JJ STRIGFELLOW

Easy 30 min Exercise Routine for Kids

For happier, healthier and more confident children

This book was professionally typeset on Reedsy.
Find out more at reedsy.com

Contents

1

Introduction

Hello, and welcome to the Easy 30 minute exercise routine for kids. My name is JJ Stringfellow. I am a father of two little boys that are ten and twelve years old. I grew up in the South. I was an athlete, a good student and had great parents that encouraged me to try hard every day. My sons and I enjoy our lives here in the Pacific Northwest. We are an active family and fill our free time with fishing, hunting, cooking, reading, writing and exercise. A balance between work and play has been an essential part of our day to day activities. Our adherence to a daily routine has been the key to our success and conquering our day.

I wrote this book because I wanted to share with you this one thing that we do together daily that has changed our lives. We participate in a daily exercise routine together. My sons and I have thrived in it. After a year working this routine into our daily lives, I can see the results in my sons and myself. The boys are happier, healthier and more confident. I have seen the changes in myself as well. My levels of energy and patience have been impacted the most. It took time, but with willingness and determination we were able to achieve our goals.

I saw my sons and I struggling in the mornings to get up and get our day started. There would be arguments over if the beds were made, who gets the first shower, what was for breakfast, what to wear for the day and what time we have to get out the door. I knew I had to get better control of our mornings. I set a schedule for the shower, made the boys get their clothes together the night before, offered either a hot or cold breakfast with only one choice for each and made 7:45am the official time getting out the door. There was something missing though. My boys do not have much interest in sports or athletics. They are active. Their bikes and scooters are ridden every day and running around the neighborhood with other kids is constant. The boys and I still seemed so sluggish in the mornings. I realized that we needed more exercise in our lives.

I wanted an activity that we could do together at home, every day. I was an avid wrestler in middle and highschool and got the Presidential physical fitness award every year in lower school. I remembered all those basic exercises and thought I could come up with a routine that was simple and easy to implement. So, I worked with my boys and we came up with a routine that is not only effective, it's easy and fun. We now have a daily routine that we do together. The boys are now doing it even when they are not home. I've seen muscle growth, weight control, better coordination, conditioning and agility. Most of all there has been a boost in confidence in themselves.

You can expect from me a clear and easy explanation of each exercise, when to do it, where to do it and how to make it fun for you and the kids. The book will have pictures of each exercise and a brief description of how to do them. We will also discuss what muscles and parts of the body each exercise is impacting so that you can talk about it during your workout routine. You will be shown the little twists and variations that make each exercise fun and a game to be enjoyed. How many mammals can you name while doing jumping jacks? Make your favorite animal sound after five sit ups. The exercise log in the back of the book will help you organize each day and record the daily accomplishments so that after some time the results and progress made can be seen. The exercises will get that heart rate and breathing rate increased and get them sweating.

Do not worry about how many push ups or sit ups are being done. Just make it fun. That is the most important factor. The results will come. The boys, like most kids, were a little hesitant at first. I had to push and encourage them every day. They got into it once they realized they were having fun and that we were all doing it together. A little competition has now been created and we are having a blast with it. The boys are waking up earlier, getting warmed up and stretching on their own. At first, I was leading the routines. Now, we schedule who is leading each day. The boys love being in charge of the routine. They are seeing who can come up with the most challenging routine and who does it the best. I have created a monster!

These exercises are easy and quick. Any parent, guardian, relative, teacher or coach can get a routine like this started. As that person in these kids' lives, we're expected to lead, encourage and motivate them. Remember to have fun at all times, follow the easy steps and you'll have success just like we did.

2

Before you begin

Getting started that first day will be the hardest part of the routine. You'll need to decide when and where you're going to work out, what exercises will be part of the routine for the day, what to wear, what items or gear you might need and who is going to struggle or do well with each exercise.

We like to begin our day with this easy routine. You might find the afternoons or evenings are better for you, or it might work better for you to mix it up. Whatever the case may be, decide when you'll be working out each day and stick with it. You do not have to do this every day. First, try every other day. When we began our routine, we would start our days Monday through Friday and take the weekends off. We are enjoying it so much that we do it every morning, every day of the week now. The morning routine works best for us, so that is what I will be discussing. By starting our day like this, we have actually accomplished something huge for the day by 7:00 am. Not many people can say that. Beds have been made. Workout routine is finished. Showers have been taken, we've gotten dressed, breakfast eaten, teeth brushed all before most folks have gotten out of bed. This is done every day. You can do it too!

Where are you going to be working out? You do not need a home gym or large area to do this. All you need is an area about the size of a yoga mat for each individual. Maybe you can pick a spot in front of the bed or couch. Just move those clothes or the coffee table out of the way. Voila! You now have your work out space. Remember that this is supposed to be easy. Put just a little effort into making a good space for the routine. A little goes a long way. The boys and I like to use our garage and backyard during the Spring and Summer months and the living room for the fall and winter months. We take turns getting the area ready each day. The boys seem to enjoy the responsibility and control they're given with this task.

We enjoy some variations on where we workout each week. Some weeks, we went to the park in the afternoon and did our workout routine there. It was fun incorporating some of the playground equipment into what we were doing. We even got other kids and parents to join us. The other kids didn't realize that it was a workout routine. They were just having fun participating with us.

Wear the basic, comfortable workout clothes for this routine. Shorts, good underwear and a t-shirt is all you really need. Socks and athletic shoes will help but they are not required. Long sleeve t-shirts, sweat shirts and sweat pants can be part of your routine. Do you want to sweat more? Throw on some layers and get that sweat on!

You will need little to no gear to begin this easy routine. Do you have carpet in your bedroom, living room or den? If you do, then you're all set. If you do not, you can use some bath towels or blankets folded up on the floor to provide a little more comfort while performing some of the exercises. Yoga mats can be purchased for around $15.

Here are some other items that you can use later in your exercises that can add comfort, a challenge and fun:

- Water bottle
- Radio
- Weights
- Timer, stopwatch, digital clock
- Elastic band
- Workout bag or storage container
- Jump rope
- Hula hoop
- Playground balls
- Cones

Your and the kid's abilities will need to be evaluated before you begin. Assess what are the physical and mental strengths and weaknesses of each individual and choose the exercises that will best suit them and what little twist or variation will make it fun for them. Keep it simple. Each kid's attitude, willingness and discipline will need to be considered. Remember to keep it easy and fun. If you are not laughing and having fun, you are doing it wrong. My boys encourage and challenge each other with each exercise now and they see who can be the funniest.

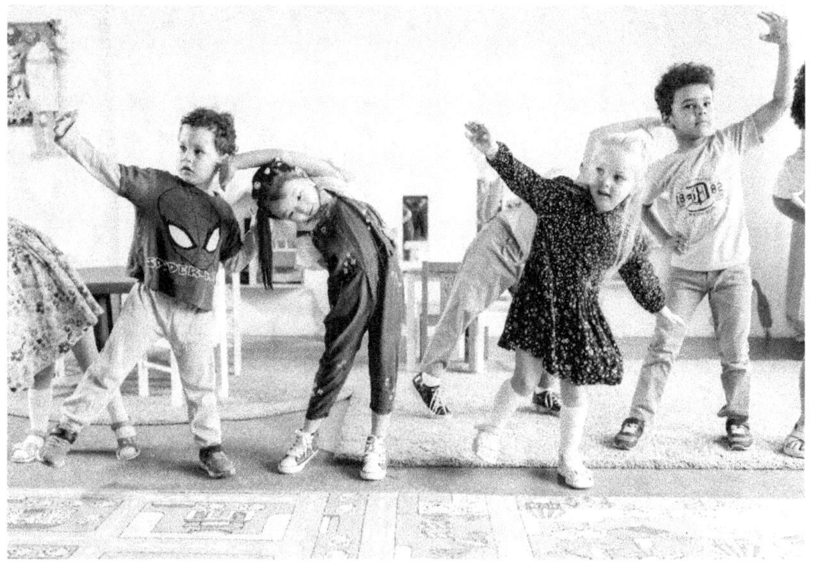

3

How to use this book

I t is up to you to decide what is going to make this fun.

This book will give you some basic and a few advanced exercises to build your routine. Select four basic exercises and one advanced. Now add a variation to the exercise that will make it fun.

I have suggested some items that will turn the exercise into a fun activity. By adding a prop, the exercise then turns into a game rather than the work that it really is.

My sons and I have added things like, name the capital of this state when we yell it out. We had also added your favorite animal sounds at the top of each sit up. It gets us laughing, exercising and thinking at the same time.

We have added combinations of exercises to change things up. An example would be, do five push ups then name your favorite mammal and make their sound. Whatever the case may be just remember to keep it fun.

4

Getting Started (5 Minutes)

To begin, set a timer for 30 minutes on your phone, watch or digital clock. It helps if you have something everyone can see. You will need to get the area ready for your routine. Start your thirty minutes.

First, take one minute to clear the floor. Move that coffee table out of the way. Pick up those clothes. Get your gear ready if you have any. Turn that radio on, get some upbeat music going and look at the workout log and choose the four basic and one advanced exercise you will be doing for the next twenty five minutes.

Second, take two minutes and warm up those muscles, tendons and ligaments that will be impacted by your exercise routine. Jumping jacks, running in place are two good warm up exercises. Start with a two minute run or walk, if you're able to. Third, take two minutes and stretch. Focus on two areas for one minute each. Start with the upper body. Stretch out arms, chest, back and neck. Then move on to the lower body. Stretch out hips, thighs and calves. These are basic stretches, so do not over think it. You are ready to begin the next twenty

9

five minutes of your easy workout routine.

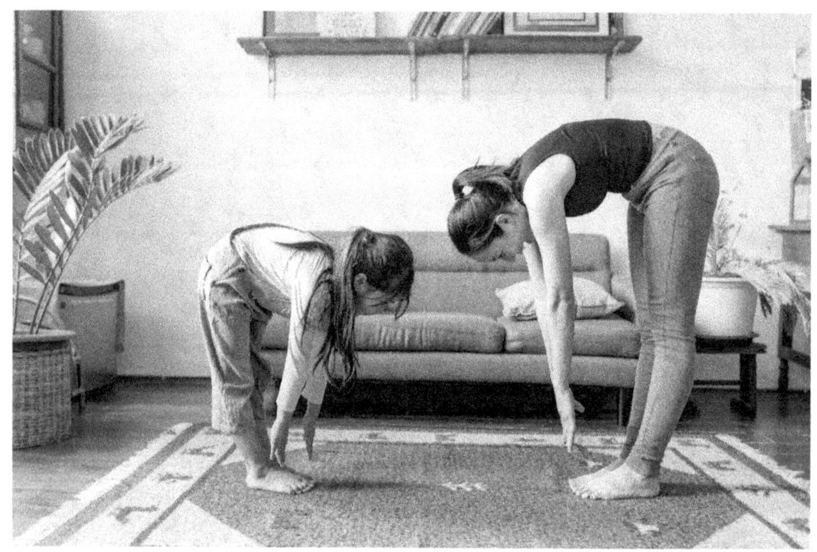

5

The Basic Exercises (20 minutes)

In this chapter, we are going to discuss each basic exercise. You will be shown proper form, what muscles and areas of the body that will be impacted and variations of each exercise that will make them enjoyable and fun.

You are going to pick four of these exercises to do for five minutes each. Do not worry about how many repetitions will be completed. Pick a number of repetitions that are doable for ten seconds. Then take a break for thirty seconds. These time periods and repetitions can be modified for each participant. This is an introduction to an exercise routine for the kids. We are not trying to break or exhaust them. This is a moment to have fun with them while teaching them a habit they can practice for the rest of their lives. Talk about the parts of the body and muscle groups that will be affected by each exercise.

1) PUSH UPS

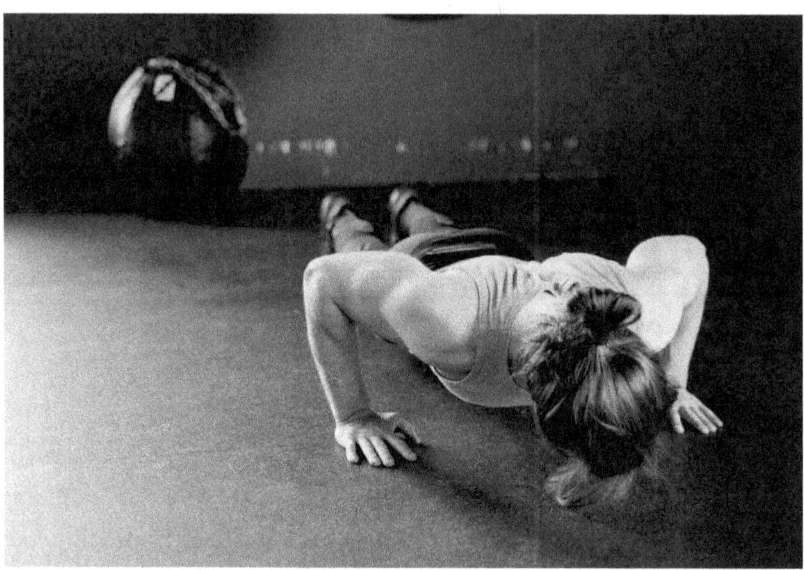

Lay face down flat on the floor. Pick your head up and look forward. Place your hands palm down, flat on the floor about shoulder width apart at the level of your chest. Have your elbows angled out away from your body. Get your feet on your tiptoes. Keep your back straight and push up. When you go back down, stop about 5 inches from the floor then push back up. Congratulations! You have just done a push up.

The areas and muscles of the body that are affected during this exercise are the chest (pectoralis), shoulders and upper arm (Deltoid, Coracobrachialis, Triceps Brachii), back and the core (abdominal muscles, serratus anterior).

VARIATIONS

Knee push ups are when instead of being on your tiptoes, your knees are down and you do the push up from there.

Full push ups are with your elbows parallel to your body and you touch your chest to the floor on the down motion of the push up.

Clappers are when you clap at the peak of the push up.

Add a ball (push up off of a playground ball)

Elevate feet and legs with a chair or bench

Elevate hands and chest with a chair or bench

One hand push up.

Push up to and arm raise.

2) SIT UPS

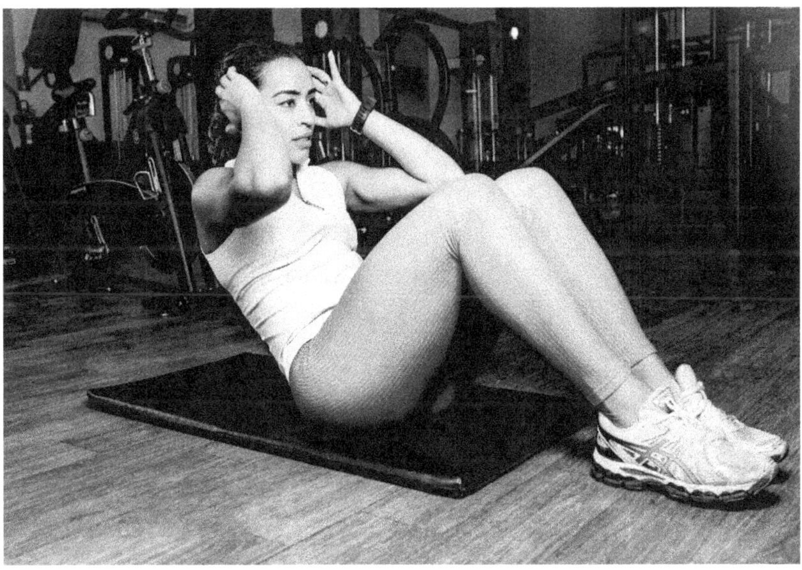

Lay on your back on the floor. Raise your knees to a forty five degree angle so that your feet are flat on the floor. Either cross your arms across your chest or put your hands behind your head. While keeping your feet flat on the floor, raise your head first, then your shoulders, then your torso off the floor and bring your chest to your knees. Congratulations. You just did a sit up.

The abdomen and core of the body are the areas affected most by sit ups. The muscles that are affected are primarily the rectus abdominis (the six pack) and the internal and external obliques. Other muscles affected are the iliopsoas (hip flexors), the rectus femoris (the front of the thigh) and some accessory muscle groups in the head, neck and shoulder area.

VARIATIONS

Crunches begin with the arms crossed across the chest or hands interlaced behind the head, knees bent at a forty five degree angle and the feet flat on the floor. Start by raising only the head and shoulders up off the floor and squeeze (crunch) those ab muscles.

Full sit ups are with the body sitting up, the legs are flat, straight out in front. Raise the arms above the head. Lean all the way back until the back touches the floor. Then raise the head, shoulders and torso up off the floor at the same time and try to touch your toes. This exercise works well with someone holding down the ankles of the one doing the exercise. Tucking feet under a couch or lip of the stairs can add some needed leverage.

Twisters are a sit up with the hands interlaced behind the head. At the top of the sit up, twist and touch the right elbow to the left knee. On the next top of the sit up, touch the left elbow to the right knee.

Flutter kicks are a crunch sit up that is held. At the top of the crunch with the legs extended straight out, hold the crunch and flutter kick (scissor motion).

3) DIPS

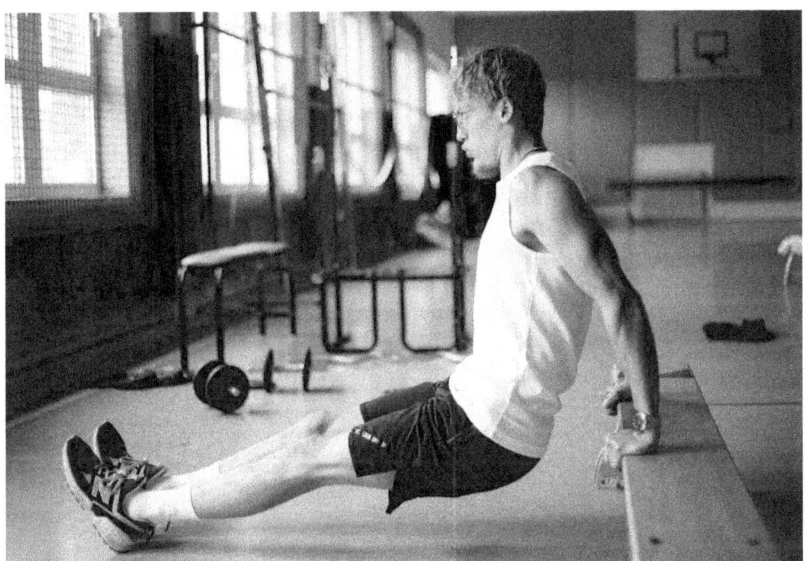

Sit on the floor with your legs together and extended in front of you. Sitting up straight, place your hands on the floor, palms flat about six inches behind you. Push up and then let your body down until your bottom touches the floor. Congratulations. You just did a dip.

The areas affected by this exercise are the back of the arms (triceps brachii), front of the shoulders (anterior deltoids), chest (pectoralis major and minor), and the back (trapezius, latissimus dorsi, teres major, levator scapulae and the rhomboids)

VARIATIONS

Chair dips are with the hands gripping the edge of a chair, legs straight out in front. Push up off the chair and lower the body till your hips are about six inches below the seat of the chair. Now push back up. Repeat.

Bench dips are with the hands gripping the edge of a bench, legs straight out in front. Push up off the bench and lower the body till your hips are about six inches below the edge of the bench seat. Now push back up. Repeat.

Stair dips dips are with the hands gripping the edge of a chair, legs straight out in front. Push up off the chair and lower the body till your hips are about six inches below the seat of the chair. Now push back up. Repeat.

4) SQUATS

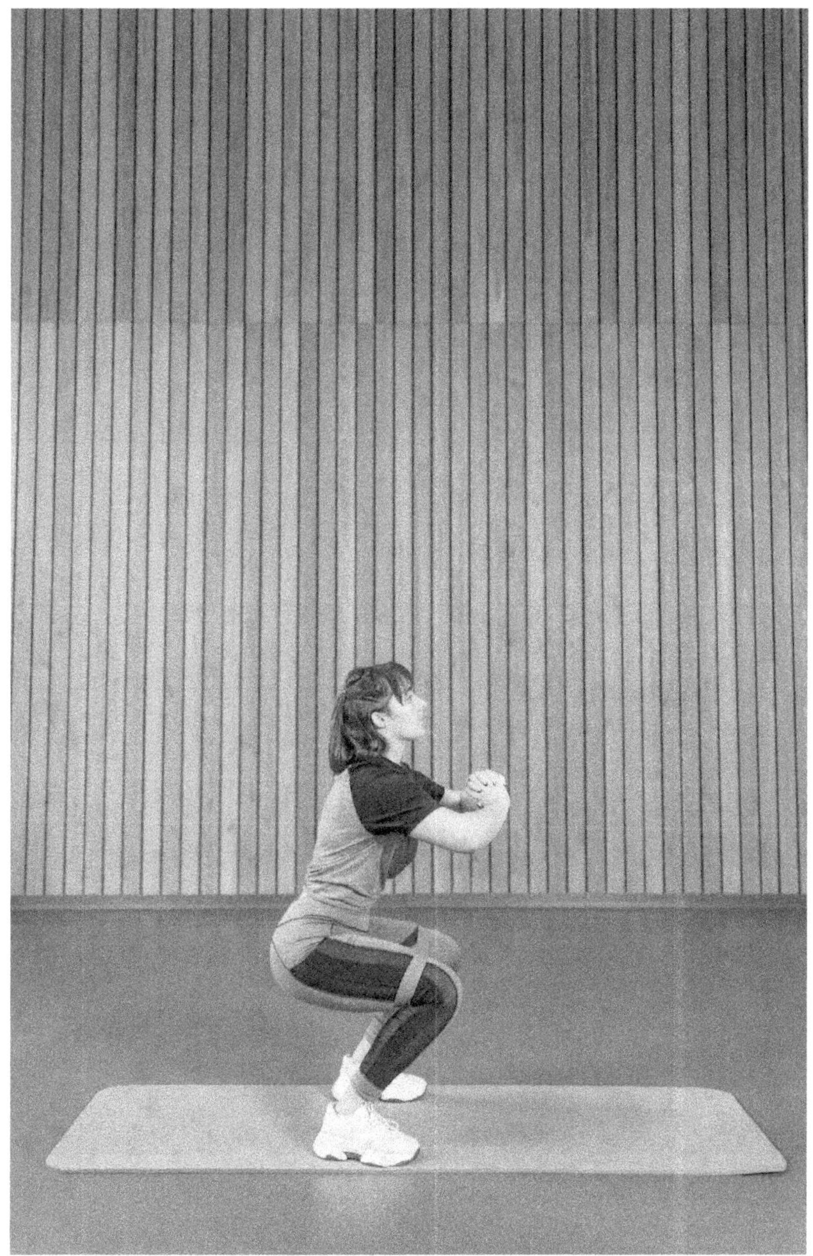

Stand with the feet shoulder width apart. Have the arms raised with the elbows pointed out at the height of the chest. Make a fist with your hands. Drop the hips until the pelvis is at the same height as the knees. Next, straighten the legs and stand back up. Repeat.

The areas of the body and the muscles affected by the squat exercise are the buttocks (gluteus maximus, minimus, medius), the front of the thigh (quadriceps), the back of the thigh (hamstrings), the groin (adductor), calves and hip flexors.

VARIATIONS

Squat with side leg raises.

Squat and finish with a jump.

5) JUMPING JACKS

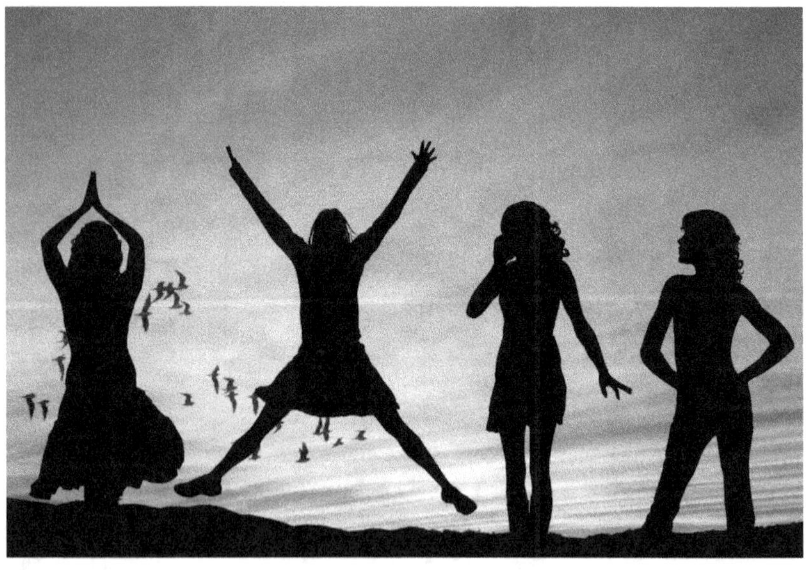

Stand with your feet together. Have your hands down by your side.

Jump and at the same time spread your feet and raise your arms and clap at the top of the jump. Jump again and bring your feet together and you arms back down to the side of your body. Repeat. Congratulations, you just did a jumping jack

The areas of the body that are affected by the jumping jack exercise are the heart, lungs, legs (glutes, hip flexors, quadriceps), the calves, shoulders and core.

6) LUNGES

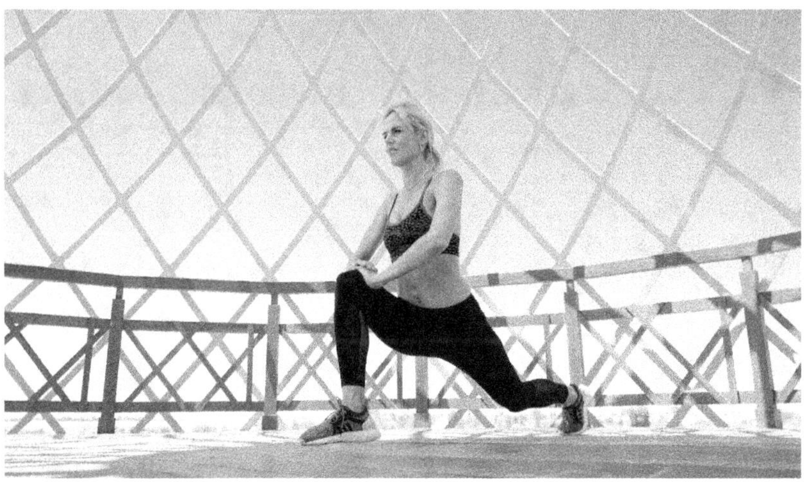

Stand up straight with your feet about shoulder width apart. Place your hands on your hips and take one full step forward with your right leg. At the same time lower your left knee and touch the floor with it. Repeat

by switching the leg that is lunging forward and the knee that touches the ground. Congratulations! You have just completed a lunge.

The areas of the body that are affected by the lunge exercise are the thighs (quadriceps, hamstrings), buttocks (gluteal muscles) and calves.

6

The Advanced Exercises (5 minutes)

I n this chapter, we are going to discuss each advanced exercise. You will be shown proper form, what muscles and areas of the body that will be impacted and variations of each exercise that will make them enjoyable and fun.

You are going to pick one of these exercises to do for five minutes. Do not worry about how many repetitions will be completed. Pick a number of repetitions that are doable for ten seconds. Then take a break for thirty seconds. These time periods and repetitions can be modified for each participant. This is an introduction to an exercise routine for the kids. We are not trying to break or exhaust them. This is a moment to have fun with them while teaching them a habit they can practice for the rest of their lives. Talk about the parts of the body and muscle groups that will be affected by each exercise.

BURPEES

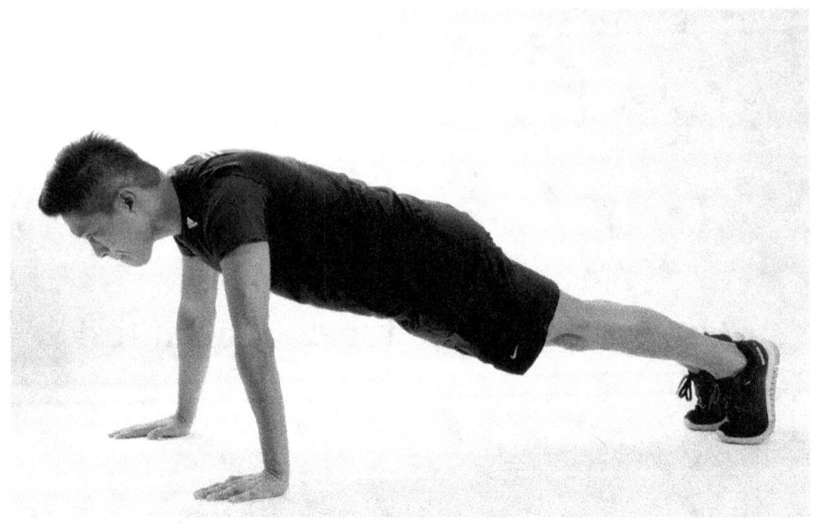

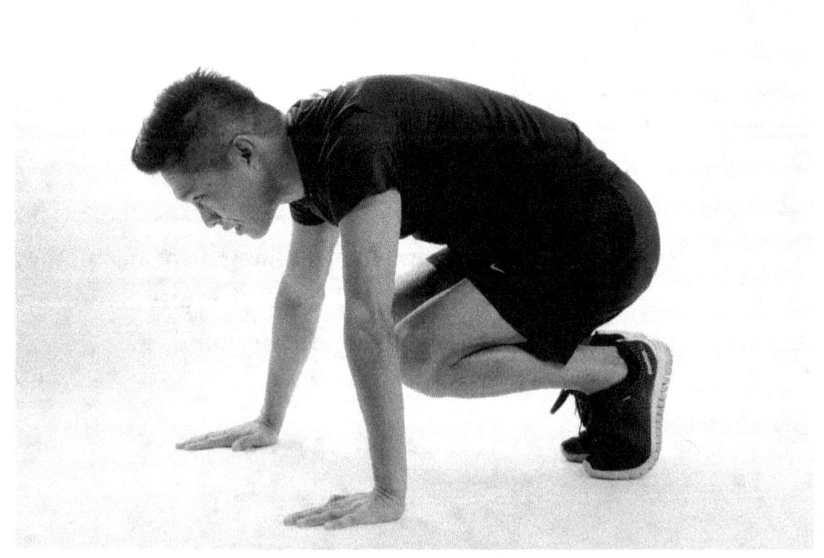

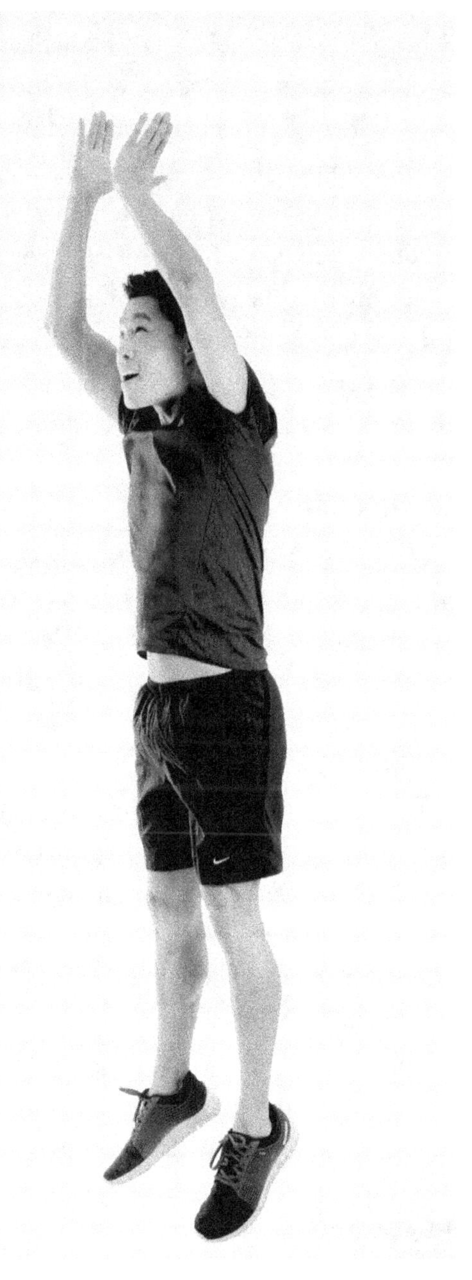

A burpee is an aerobic exercise that has two components. It is a push up, then a jump. Lay face down on the floor. Do a full push up. At the top of the push up, bring your feet up to your hands. Stand straight up and jump in the air. After you land, return to the push up position and complete another pushup. Repeat as many times as you can for 30 seconds, then take a break for 30 seconds.

The areas of the body and muscles that are affected by a burpee are the legs (glutes, hip flexors, quadriceps), chest (pectoralis), shoulders and upper arm (Deltoid, Coracobrachialis, Triceps Brachii), back and the core (abdominal muscles, serratus anterior).

HIGH KNEE

A high knee exercise combines a run in place with an exaggerated lifting of the knee at the top of the exercise.

The areas of the body and muscles affected by a high knee exercise are the thighs (quads, hamstrings), calves and buttocks (glutes).

CLIMBERS

The climber exercise is a push up that is held at the top of the exercise. Start by laying face down. Do a push up with your hands about shoulder width apart. Keep your toes touching the floor. Bring a knee up to the center of your body and then switch legs quickly. Repeat quickly alternating between both legs as you hold the push up. Congratulations! You just did a climber.

The areas and muscles of the body that are affected by the climber exercise are the abdominal muscles, triceps, shoulder muscles, serratus anterior and chest muscles

PLANKS

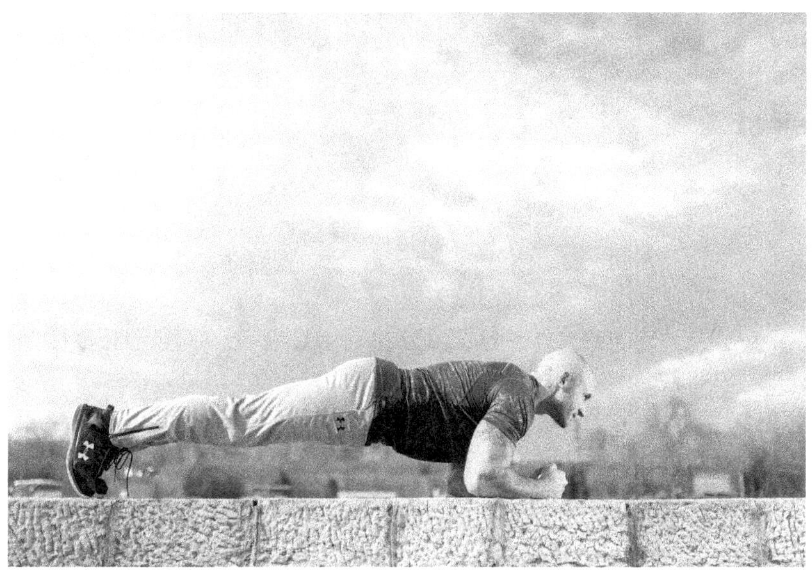

Plank exercises are accomplished by laying face down on the floor. With your elbows at shoulder level, place all of your weight on your forearms and tip toes. Your body should be straight. Congratulations! You have now done a plank.

The areas and muscles of the body that are affected by the plank exercise are the front abs (rectus abdominis), the side abs (obliques), the belly (transverse abdominis) and the buttocks (glutes).

VARIATIONS

Plank with an arm raise is accomplished by doing a plank and raising one arm straight up from the floor. Hold for five seconds. Go back down and repeat with the opposite arm.

Plank with a leg raise is accomplished by doing a plank and lifting one leg straight up from the floor. Hold for five seconds. Go back down with your leg and repeat with the opposite leg.

7

A day in the life of an active routine

The boys and I get up at 6:00 am everyday including the weekends. We wake up, and change into our work out clothes. Thomas selects good underwear and a sweatshirt and sweatpants. He likes to get heated up and perspire. Rex and I put on good underwear, athletic shorts and a t-shirt. We meet in our living room, move the coffee table out of the way and push the couch back to give ourselves a little more space.

Rex is going to lead the exercise routine today. We have a large digital clock set on the coffee table so that we can all see it. He turns the radio on so we can listen to rock and roll while we exercise. He hits the button starting the timer and we're off. He has us start by doing jumping jacks for one minute followed by one minute of running in place. This gets our heart rate and breathing rate elevated. Our muscles, ligaments and tendons are now warmed up and ready to stretch.

Rex leads us in some basic stretches for the next two minutes. We twist left and right to stretch out our backs. We roll our necks around. We grab our elbow with the opposite hand and pull the arm across our chest stretching out our shoulders. We stand with our legs spread a little further than shoulder width apart and lean to each side stretching out our groins, hips and buttocks. Next we sit down with our legs straight out in front of us and do some toe touches. While in this position we twist and stretch out our backs again.

Rex gives us a quick run down of the exercises we'll be doing today. "Ok, guys. Today we will be doing push ups, sit ups, dips and squats as our basic exercises. Then we will be doing burpees for our advanced exercises."

As our routine leader, Rex has come up with the little variations that are going to make it fun and challenging. He had previously gone into one of their old toy chests and found three kazoos. He tells us that for the time that we are actually doing push ups, we are to sing the Happy Birthday song into the kazoo and we have to do it in unison. Hilarity begins for the next five minutes. We start by laying down and getting our bodies in the push up exercise. He starts with the down push up and we all start singing into the kazoo. Not only are we getting a workout with the push ups but we are having to control our breathing while exercising and singing at the same time. We take a short break. Then we start another round of push ups but his time we have to sing the abc song into the kazoo.

The sit ups are next for five minutes. We start by sitting on the floor with our legs bent at a forty five degree angle and our toes underneath the edge of the couch. Rex lets us know that we will be doing a sit up with a twist. At the top of the sit up we are to make our favorite animal noise. Thomas picks a dog. I pick a cow, and Rex picks a crow. He starts the sit ups and it now sounds like a farm in our living room. Our muscles are getting tired from the exercise and also the laughter as we find enjoyment in each of our animal sounds. We each get in around twenty sit ups before we take a break for thirty seconds. You can see the wheels turning in Rex's head as he comes up with the next twist. For the next round of sit ups we have to make the animal noise of the others in the group, switching it up at the top of each sit up.

For the next five minutes we do dips and use the couch to elevate our upper body with our feet on the floor, stretched out straight in front of us. At the top of each dip, we are to name a state and the others have to name the capital of that state. This has proven to be a challenge and only got easier as we all learned the capital of each state.

Rex has us do squats for five minutes for our last basic exercise. He has each of us take a playground ball. At the top of each squat we are to dribble the ball five times then squat again. Since this is the last of the basic exercises, we are to do squats for one minute, then take a thirty second break and then begin again. The squat gets the thighs and the buttocks burning. The dribbling of the ball helps us with coordination and balance.

Burpees are going to be our advanced and final exercise for five minutes. We begin laying face down and do a push up. We bring our knees up to our chest and then leap into the air, then back down into a pushup. Rex's twist on the burpee is for him to call out a simple multiplication problem and then we are to answer. "Two times two is.." and we call out "four". We do burpees for one minute then rest for thirty seconds.

We have now done our routine for thirty minutes. We are tired but energized for the day. Rex leads us in some simple stretches as we cool down and we get to talking about the farm animal noises we each choose. Thomas and I begin to think of what little twist we are going to incorporate into our routine when it comes time for us to lead.

Showers are being taken. The boys are getting dressed for school. Breakfast is being eaten, and we are out the door by 7:45am. The boys and I are happy and healthy and i can see that they are beaming with confidence as we go and conquer our day.

8

Conclusion

By now you have been introduced to some basic and a few advanced exercises that you can use to build your daily routine. As you move forward, your adherence with just getting in there and trying will make all the difference. Taking the time to assess your kids capabilities and learning what they think of as fun will lead to your success with this routine. The boys and I have become closer. We love challenging each other and we especially love making each other laugh. Screwing up the exercises has been a fun part of it as well. The boys have benefited from seeing me be vulnerable and trying their twists on the routine no matter how silly it seems.

I hope that you have enjoyed my book and have gotten some useful tips on how to go about not only getting started but also on how to have fun while doing it. You can be the class clown and the leader of this exercise routine. Remember. Use your imagination and always practice patience when dealing with kids, and above all, have fun while you are doing it. If you feel like this book has helped you in any way, please leave a positive review and also recommend it to your family and friends.